INTERMITTENT FASTING

Complete Beginner's Guide To Lose Weight, Burn Fat And Stay Healthy Through Intermittent Fasting

ELIZABETH WELLS

TABLE OF CONTENTS

Free Bonus
The Best Foods To Eat On A Ketogenic Diet

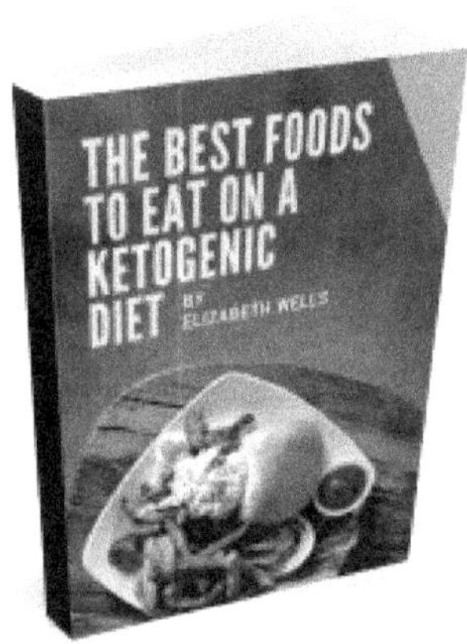

Discover the best foods to eat on a ketogenic diet. You'll learn the different food groups that you should eat to follow the keto diet correctly and start improving your health right now.

Go to **www.eepurl.com/cUqOlH** to download the guide for free.

Introduction

Thank you for purchasing *Intermittent Fasting: Complete Beginner's Guide To Lose Weight, Burn Fat And Stay Healthy Through Intermittent Fasting*

There is plenty of information on the Internet about Intermittent Fasting (IF), but the purpose of this book is to give the reader the knowledge needed to begin an IF diet tomorrow if that is the goal. This Introduction will briefly summarize the major bullet points of IF. It will also explain the topics covered in each chapter in case you'd like to skip ahead and have a peak. So, let's jump right into the shallow end of the pool.

What is Intermittent Fasting?

A fast is a period in which one abstains from food and drink. Human beings have been fasting since the beginning of the species. This may have been a practical concern: all of the wildebeest, moose, reindeer, or other game had migrated to a watering hole a hundred miles away (along with all the fish, apparently). Fasting may also have cultural and religious connotations, that is, fasting deliberately for a purpose that has nothing to do with the actual availability of food. **Intermittent Fasting is the purposeful restriction of food and drinks during a specified period to encourage weight loss.** It is called "intermittent" because one is eating intermittently; long periods of fasting are punctuated by a period of eating and drinking. When one isn't eating, one is fasting.

Intermittent Fasting has become increasingly popular due to its health benefits and its ability to rapidly change body composition. There are different types of Intermittent Fasting, which will be discussed in a minute, but the most common form of Intermittent Fasting involves eating during a specified window each day and dieting for the hours outside of that window. For example, a dieter may decide that they like to have their last bite to eat no later than 7 PM. Well, if your Intermittent Fasting regimen is a 16/8 split (16 hours of fasting and 8 hours of eating), then all of your meals would have to be taken in an 8-hour window. In this case, you would be eating between 11 AM and 7 PM and fasting during the hours outside of this window.

One of the primary benefits of Intermittent Fasting is that it can help anyone achieve their goals, whether they are Don the Forklift Driver trying to lose a little bit of weight, or Larry, an Amateur Bodybuilder attempting to lower his body fat below 10 percent. Intermittent Fasting has not only been shown to be effective at helping beginners lose fat, often much more quickly and consistently than other diets, but because it is tapping into the inherent physiology of the human body, dieters who utilize Intermittent Fasting tend to keep the weight off and to feel healthier and more energetic even though they are actually fasting for several hours in the day.

The two main types of Intermittent Fasting are called Whole Day (or Alternate Day) Fasting and Time-Restricted Feeding. The names pretty much tell you what they are, but Alternate Day Fasting means that you are not eating anything for the entire day and the only thing you are taking in is water. Time-restricted feeding means that your eating or "feeding" is restricted to a certain window of the day, like 8 hours, 10 hours, 4 hours, etc. Most people who try Intermittent Fasting commonly take advantage of Time-restricted Feeding (TRF) as this works well for individuals who are attempting to shed fat while building muscle. It also works well for folks who have busy schedules and for whom fasting an entire day might be difficult. Both approaches to Intermittent Fasting will be discussed.

The *Intermittent Fasting: Complete Beginner's Guide To Lose Weight, Burn Fat And Stay Healthy Through Intermittent Fasting* is designed to help anyone interested in losing weight or lowering their body fat find the right approach to meet their goals. With that end in mind, this book will explain (in often excruciating detail!) how Intermittent Fasting works and why. This will be accomplished in six approachable, readable chapters. At the end of each chapter are *Summary Points* that reiterate the major concepts of the chapter for efficient understanding and information processing.

The book will also help the reader achieve fat loss by offering suggested splits, workout routines, and offering recipes. *Chapter 2 (Alternate Day Fasting vs. Time-restricted Feeding)* presents a detailed explanation of the two main types of Intermittent Fasting and addresses why someone might choose one over the other. *Chapter 3 (Setting Goals)* will help the reader identify what their goals are in their diet so they can choose the split that works for them and monitor their progress. *Chapter 4 (Intermittent Fasting for Weight Loss)* is designed for the person attempting to shed those additional pounds, while *Chapter 5 (Intermittent Fasting for Bodybuilding)* is tailored to the bodybuilder whose primary goal is lowering body fat while preserving muscle.

Chapter 6 addresses the Frequently Asked Questions people generally have when it comes to Intermittent Fasting, and there are many. Very, very many. You might want to take a quick peek at Chapter 6 to familiarize yourself with the sort of questions potential IFers generally have. But we begin with Chapter 1, where we take a long trip back in time where we find an early human hunting his dinner with a flint-tipped javelin.

Chapter 1
But... Breakfast is the Most Important Meal of the Day!

For humans living 10,000 years ago, it wasn't. It arguably wasn't even important just 1000 years ago. Indeed, the term "breakfast" suggests that the first meal of the day broke a period of fasting, and these periods of fasting, often for religious purposes, were considered normal in pre-modern times. Conventions about when meals should be eaten are modern inventions. In Europe in the Middle Ages, people ate two meals: dinner and supper. Dinner was actually eaten early in the day, not in the evening. The word dinner, from French *disner*, actually meant "break fast." This dinner would not have been consumed at dawn, when people generally first got up to work in the fields – or whatever Middle Age serfs and peasants would have been doing at dawn. But after several hours of work, when the sun was up, and people could see what they were eating... *Hey, don't eat that! That's milord's favorite hunting hound!* No artificial lighting, remember? The evening meal, consumed after all the work for the day had been done, was called supper. So dinner was breakfast. ...and supper was dinner. Confused? Don't be. The important point here is that skipping "breakfast," or what we call breakfast, isn't anything new.

In fact, prehistoric human beings would have been engaged in a similar practice as their cousins of the Middle Ages - eating fewer meals during the day over a shorter period. Our early ancestors of the prehistoric period would not only lack our modern sense of time and the idea that certain things should always be done at certain times of the day - like eating for example. They would not have farmed so they probably would not have been able to eat "breakfast" (that is, the modern breakfast) even if they wanted to.

There's a show that comes on television called *Naked and Afraid,* where the contestants have to try to survive in the wilderness for 21 days without any clothes, and with only their wits to carry them through those three weeks. They have to hunt, fish, eat bugs and worms, make fire, find shelter, etc. all without modern technology. One thing one notices right away is not only that it's hard out there for a naked human with no microwave or cell phone, but that our perceptions around food are very much dictated by culture and, by extension, technology. The first thing the contestants on *Naked and Afraid* do in the morning is not eat "breakfast." How can they? That would mean spending six hours collecting enough bugs to form a breakfast or four or five hours fishing. Perhaps building a trap to catch a rat or some other small creature of the forest. They could try hunting bigger game, but that would mean they would have to create some sort of sturdy weapons, like a spear or javelin, first, wouldn't it? That's another six to 12 hours. You get the idea. Breakfast is really a modern invention, a tasty one, but definitely modern.

Of course, there are benefits to eating breakfast.

Just like Smokey the Bear taught me that it's important to prevent forest fires, a leprechaun lets me in on the fact that I am supposed to eat some sugary, dyed marshmallow charms first thing in the morning, so I have enough energy to ignore everything that I am supposed to be learning in school. Don't get me wrong. I am not anti-breakfast, but it is important that we examine where many of our beliefs about food come from. If you are just starting out in fitness and your primary goal is losing weight, an important step for you –perhaps the most important –is to examine your eating habits, both in terms of quantity and quality of food, and figuring out how you will make Intermittent Fasting work for you. In reality, it's easy once you realize how your body is supposed to process food and how Intermittent Fasting essentially taps into this evolutionary mechanism to force your body to shed fat.

The Physiology of Intermittent Fasting

Intermittent Fasting is unique as far as diets go because it makes use of the body's natural way of processing food. When we eat, excess food is stored for later use, when we're fasting. Fatty acids are stored as triglycerides in adipose tissue (fat) in various regions of our body. Molecules of glucose are strung together to form a large molecule called glycogen that is stored in muscle. Fat is nothing more than a convenient store of energy molecules that our body can access later when it needs to. The problems that most people have with fat is that prolonged binge eating, in which we overwhelm our bodies with massive amounts of food, actually causes our body to lower its metabolic rate, making it harder for us to mobilize fat when we later need to. Another thing caloric excess does, and this is significant, is it causes our bodies to become resistant to insulin. Insulin is a hormone that promotes the absorption of glucose into the cells, allowing glucose to be metabolized and used for energy. Insulin resistance is also, by definition, Type 2 Diabetes, so the relatively modern (in evolutionary terms) practice of eating large amounts of food for prolonged periods of the day actually makes us insulin resistant and leads us on the road towards Type 2 Diabetes. Type 2 Diabetes is associated with a host of unwanted morbidities, and an at-length discussion of them exceeds the scope of this work. Suffice it to say that heart disease, stroke, retinopathy, neuropathy, and all of the other conditions that diabetes puts you at risk for is something that you want to steer clear of.

Long-term energy reserves	Molecule	Purpose
Adipose Tissue (Fat)	Triglyceride	Used by muscle and cardiac tissue as fuel
Glycogen (in Muscle and Liver)	Glycogen	Used as an energy source

The point here is that the body stores fatty acids and glucose for later use because it expects our bodies to have periods when we are not eating. Do not forget Reginald, the Middle Ages peasant, or Dominic, the guy from New Jersey who has to spend seven hours trying to catch a fish with a spear on

Naked and Afraid. We may have been taught as children that breakfast was the most important meal of the day and I don't want to say that it isn't. I mean, I want to, but I won't. Breakfast may be "important" in a modern world of electric light and cars and 8 to 5s or 7 to 5s, whatever. But eating three large meals every day is probably why many of us are obese. I can attest that nearly all of the contestants on *Naked and Afraid* were looking pretty svelte at the end of the 21 days.

In simpler terms, Intermittent Fasting works by triggering your body to mobilize its stores of fat when you are fasting. It's pretty straightforward. When you rise in the morning and go through your daily routine, your body will naturally have some energy requirements so it will tap into the fat. Because you have not been eating for how many hours of the night, your metabolic rate will be fairly high, encouraging your body to quickly and efficiently mobilize that fat. This is the first trigger of weight loss. Let's say that it's Saturday, your day off, and after a few hours on the computer, you plan to head to the gym at 11 AM and have your first IF meal of the day at 12. You might be concerned that you won't have any energy for your workout since you've already been up for several hours without food. Well, that's what the glycogen is for. The body will mobilize glycogen to release glucose for those short bursts of action while working out. Any other energy needs, like half an hour on the treadmill or in the pool, for example, can easily be handled by the body with fatty acids mobilized from your fat stores. What's the point? Rather than your body deriving energy for your workout from the food you ate that morning, it actually will tap into your supply of fat and glycogen and use that for energy, not only causing you to lose weight in the form of fat but also increasing your metabolic rate and making you more sensitive to insulin.

Because Intermittent Fasting is piggybacking off of the body's natural system of storing fat and glycogen, and mobilizing them later, following this eating regimen confers a host of benefits. A recent study has shown that Intermittent Fasting, as a standalone diet and compared to other diets, is better at triggering weight loss, improves cardiovascular health, decreases cancer risk, has neuroprotective effects, and increases lifespan. This information is not new, the Ancient Greeks wrote about the benefits of fasting more than 2000 years ago. A gentleman named Luigi Cornaro (no relation to Mario Brothers) who lived in Italy in the 15th century survived to the age of 102 at a time when the average life expectancy in Europe was between 30 and 40. When he was in his eighties, he was asked to write down his daily routine so that others could get an idea of why he was living so much longer than other people in Europe at the time. He wrote a book called (in English) *Discourses on a Temperate Life*, in which he reported that he ate 350 grams of food a day and drank almost half a liter of wine. Everyday. If we assume that 50 grams of Luigi's diet came from fat and the rest from carbohydrates and protein, that means that Luigi was getting about 1650 calories a day, not including the wine. Strange as it may seem, Luigi's case was one of the first on record in which a link was made between diet (in this case, calorie restriction) and increased lifespan.

"So you're telling me that our prehistoric ancestors all lived to 102 because they were eating better then than we are now?" Absolutely not. Our prehistoric ancestors mostly died by thirty, but that had nothing to do with diet and had everything to do with sharing the neighborhood with elephants, a rhinoceros, and other wild animals who probably killed them before they would have reaped any benefits from their Intermittent Fasting diet. Fortunately for you, reader, being trampled by an elephant isn't something you have to worry about so you can spend your time reading (and thinking) about insulin instead...

The Role of Insulin in Intermittent Fasting

...Which leads us to the subject of Insulin. Anyone who reads fitness or bodybuilding magazines, or follows any bodybuilding or health-related channels on YouTube, is familiar with insulin as a hot topic in the bodybuilding world. Insulin is very actively discussed these days, not so much regarding its negative associations –the link with Diabetes, for example –but for its potential uses. It is a hormone that can be manipulated by diet and exercise. It's not as hokey as it sounds. Nutritionists and personal trainers are studying insulin and the effects that this hormone has on the body to help bodybuilders and fitness enthusiasts realize their full potential in the industry. We have already learned that insulin helps get glucose into our cells and that Intermittent Fasting increases insulin sensitivity. But so what?

One of the reasons why Intermittent Fasting works so well as a diet is because it helps the body to utilize and store energy more efficiently. This means a few different things. One is that, essentially, the body is using the form of energy that it prefers to meet its energy requirements. The preferred energy source for the body at most time is glucose or sugar. So if you have glucose in your bloodstream, from a recent meal, for example, then your body will use that. So having a workout after you've had breakfast will create a situation where your body will be using that energy source to meet its needs during the workout, not burning fat, which is what you want and which is also what the body is expecting. Remember, the reason why we store fat and glycogen in the first place is that our body is expecting to have periods where it needs to operate without any glucose in the bloodstream. When our body is using these stores for energy early in the day, it is actually operating efficiently by using the stores that it was expecting to use rather than being confused by all the maple syrup that you put on your pancakes for breakfast. This latter case would be inefficient because your body thinks that it should be mobilizing your adipose tissue to release fatty acids for energy when all of A sudden it gets smacked in the face with all of the sugar that you consumed for breakfast. Your body actually has to expend energy to digest and process food. So when you have a breakfast meal before a workout, your body is both expending energy to digest that meal at the same time that it is trying to meet the energy requirements associated with your workout.

I think you can see why this is inefficient. In this situation, where you are working out on a full stomach, your body is being forced to do multiple things at once. It's digesting the food that you've eaten, it's attempting to use some of the glucose that has entered the bloodstream from that meal for energy, it may be mobilizing some of your glycogen stores for energy as well and,if you had a large meal, it might be trying to store some of those fatty acids as fat. The ideal situation for fat loss, or just for a smoothly operating system (your body), is for you to actually not have eaten before your workout, or at least to have your meal spaced far enough from your workout that your body is not confused and can use its preferred energy source.

Another dimension to this is, since our goal is fat loss, we actually want the body to be operating efficiently not only regarding how it is mobilizing our fat and glycogen stores but also in how it stores them. The ideal situation is that fat and glycogen will be mobilized for energy during a workout. After a workout and we have a meal, our body replenishes the glycogen stores for the next time we need a burst of energy. Also, our body is using the meal that we have eaten to help recover from the workout, rather than storing the energy from the meal as fat. That is a system that is operating efficiently.

Insulin sensitivity is closely tied to all of this. As mentioned above, Intermittent Fasting increases the body's sensitivity to insulin. Eating when you're not hungry, binge eating, or any dietary habit that tends to cause hyperglycemia (increased glucose in the bloodstream) will reduce insulin sensitivity. Reduced insulin sensitivity not only shifts the body towards fat storage, but it is also the first step toward developing Type 2 Diabetes.

Summary Points

1. Our human ancestors would not have consumed breakfast.
2. Intermittent Fasting replicates a human being's natural dietary state, that is, relatively short periods of eating punctuated by longer periods where we are not eating.
3. Intermittent Fasting works by mobilizing fat and glycogen from the body's own stores for

energy during a fasting period, rather than using circulating glucose from a recent meal.

4. Observations from as early as the Classical Period demonstrated that periods of fasting and reduced caloric intake were associated with longevity and other health benefits.

5. We know that at least some of the benefits of Intermittent Fasting have to do with efficient storage of energy and increased sensitivity to insulin.

Chapter 2
Whole-Day Fasting vs. Time-Restricted Feeding

This chapter will address the two main types of Intermittent Fasting and explain why one individual might choose one type over the other. What's great about Intermittent Fasting is that anyone can achieve their goals with this regimen, regardless of what their goals are. We will address setting goals in the next chapter, but this chapter will provide you with the understanding of IF types that will aid you in tailoring Intermittent Fasting to your specific goals. In reality, Intermittent Fasting is pretty straightforward once you understand what it is and there really isn't too much tailoring required.

The two main types of Intermittent Fasting are Whole-Day Fasting (also called Alternate Day Fasting or ADF) and Time-Restricted Feeding (TRF). Alternate Day Fasting involves not eating anything at all over a 24-hour period. One only eats the day after the 24-hour period of fasting. Technically, during the day of eating, the hours in which one eats are not limited, though the individual may choose to eat during a shorter window, essentially combining Alternate Day Fasting with the other type of

Intermittent Fasting: Time-restricted Feeding. Fasting for more than 48 hours is referred to as Prolonged Fasting and is usually not considered a type of Intermittent Fasting since it is not really intermittent. Remember, this diet is called *Intermittent* Fasting because periods of fasting are broken up by periods of eating and a fast of 120 hours, for example, is long enough that we generally wouldn't consider the eating after it to be intermittent.

The other main type of Intermittent Fasting is Time-restricted Feeding. This type is popular among bodybuilding and fitness enthusiasts because it allows them to lose fat relatively quickly while preserving their muscle mass. The human body has several adaptations that make fasting not only sustainable for humans but preferable at times, and one could argue that Time-restricted feeding provides the best balance between losing weight and still being able to meet one's responsibilities, like having a job, family, etc. Of course, the weight loss in Time-restricted feeding may not be as rapid as in Alternate Day Fasting, but we're jumping the gun a little bit here, so let's start by delving into Time-Restricted Feeding a little bit more.

In Time-Restricted Feeding, the individual fasts for certain periods during the day (most of the day) and eats during a specified window. This eating window is the same every day. Pretty simple, right? The idea is that when you are fasting, you are using fat stores in the form of adipose tissue for most of the body's energy requirements and tapping into the muscle's glycogen stores for short bursts of energy, during a workout, for example. The individual can tailor the window of eating to meet their needs, although this book will specifically address the most popular choices: 4 hours, 8 hours, and 10 hours. The most popular choice for eating window in Time-restricted Feeding is 8 hours, and this regimen is called a 16/8 protocol, that is, 16 hours of fasting and 8 hours of eating. This fasting period is not quite as restrictive as it sounds as the 16 hours includes sleep. Therefore, daytime hours of fasting are closer to 7-9 hours.

Pros and Cons of Alternate Day Fasting

The primary benefit of Alternate Day Fasting is that it has been clinically shown to cause very rapid weight loss. It is not difficult to understand why. The reason why Intermittent Fasting triggers weight loss is due to our body being forced to mobilize fat when we are not eating, so if we are not eating for a whole day, that's a whole day of our body churning that fat. This type of diet would cause more rapid weight loss than a diet that merely targets what we're eating because even if we're eating in smaller portions, we're essentially still eating so our body is not targeting body fat to the same degree that it would during a whole day fast. Added to this is the reality that many overweight and obese individuals have metabolic concerns. If you are on a diet that is restricting your calories, or even just cutting out most of the fat or carbohydrates, the unfortunate reality may be that your metabolic rate is so low that you still aren't really attacking fat in the same way you would if you were fasting for the whole day. Obese people often have to severely restrict their caloric intake to see results in a reasonable amount of time.

Another benefit of Alternate Day Fasting is that it is a straightforward, simple diet to adopt since the primary modification being made is simply not eating for a day. You don't have to think about meal timing; you don't even have to pay attention to any of the excruciating details about macros (macronutrients). All you're doing is not eating for a day. Now, obviously, this diet works better if you are also paying attention to what you are eating. As the goal in this book is to help you reach your dieting goals, whether they are weight loss or specifically fat loss (lowered BF percentage), we will present meal breakdowns and recipes in chapters 4 and 5 that will make it easier to adopt this type of IF or the other type, Time-Restricted Feeding.

Of course, Alternate Day Fasting is not easy. If it were easy, everyone would do it. For someone who is used to eating fast food from sunup to sundown, not eating for a whole day is a pretty big step, even if it is just one step. Alternate Day Fasting assumes a fair measure of discipline and dedication. Alternate Day Fasting also assumes that the individual is healthy enough to not eat for an entire day. So, before starting this diet, it would be important to consult your doctor or healthcare provider.

Pros and Cons of Time-restricted Feeding

Time-restricted Feeding refers to eating during a certain window in the day and fasting for the period outside of this window. The advantages of Time-restricted Feeding are manifold. Time-restricted Feeding has been clinically shown to cause rapid and lasting fat loss, less muscle loss, and increased insulin sensitivity and glycogen storage resulting in more efficient sugar regulation and improved cardiovascular health. A recent study has shown that periods of fasting during the day, in addition to the benefits already mentioned, also confers neuroprotective effects, decreases cancer risk, and may increase lifespan. Of course, this last study was conducted on rats, but we also have the evidence of our friend Luigi Cornaro who managed to live to the age of 102 in the Middle Ages, when the average life expectancy was about 35.

Another major "pro" of Time-restricted Feeding is that, as a diet, it may be more amenable to the lives of most people compared to Alternate Day Fasting because one should not have any trouble meeting their daily responsibilities on this diet. Think about it this way: if the typical American adopts this type of diet and eats for 12 hours in the day, he's basically just cutting out four of those hours – skipping breakfast, for example. That may not be easy, but it would represent less of a life-modification than not eating for an entire day.

The major drawback of Time-restricted Feeding has already been mentioned. Skipping breakfast. Yes, most of us in this country have been taught that breakfast is the most important meal of the day and the idea of not eating breakfast may be difficult to wrap your head around. Technically, no one is telling you that you have to skip breakfast on a 16/8 protocol of Time-restricted Feeding. If Captain Crunch means that much to you, you can start your eight-hour window in the morning, at 8AM for example. Thing is, you would have to have your last meal by 4PM. That is, swallow that bite of food before the clock strikes 4. Other than that (getting used to skipping a meal, like breakfast), there really aren't too many drawbacks to Time-restricted Feeding.

Caloric Restriction

So technically, Caloric Restriction isn't a *type* of Intermittent Fasting, but it is important to be discussed here because we will be addressing it in the next three chapters. Most diets are based on the idea of caloric restriction. All that means is eating fewer calories during the day. Instead of that McRib from McDonald's (do they still make those? The McRib *was* always my weakness), you have a small chicken salad with a light dressing (or no dressing at all). A salad has fewer calories than a McRib; it also has less fat, carbohydrates, and cholesterol. Low-fat diets are also caloric restriction diets because fat has more calories per gram than other types of micronutrients (see the itty-bitty table below):

Macronutrient	Calories per gram
Protein	4
Carbohydrates	4
Fat	9
Alcohol	7

See that? Fat has more than twice as many calories per gram than any of the other macronutrients except alcohol, so a high-fat diet (the typical American diet) is also going to put the average person in a daily caloric excess. So, if you should be getting 2000 calories a day (based on your BMI and your activity level), then a high-fat diet can easily put you at 3000 calories a day. Most of those extra calories will be stored as fat, so most diets try to target this unsuitability of fat by cutting most of the fat out of your diet. It also makes logical sense to cut fat out of your diet since the goal of most dieters is to shed fat. Some diets also (or specifically) target carbohydrates (sugar) because a feature of the modern Western diet compared to the diets of our prehistoric ancestors is the massive amount of sugar that we consume. Our ancestors' primary source of sugar was in the form of plant starch (like fruits and vegetables), and their diets would have been higher in protein and, well, fat. We actually drink liquid sugar in the form of soda, and as our body converts excess glucose into fatty acids and stores it as fat, a diet that targets carbs would help us to reduce fat storage.

But I think it's easy to see how Intermittent Fasting has an advantage over even a low carb Paleo type of diet. Intermittent Fasting is not only reducing caloric intake or reducing fat storage; it actually is removing fat from our bodies and making our body more efficient in the way that it handles calories. There is, naturally, an overlap between Caloric Restriction and Intermittent Fasting though, technically Caloric Restriction is not an automatic component of IF. A competitive bodybuilding or fitness competitor might adopt a Time-restricted Feeding diet while technically not being particularly calorie-restricted. In other words, on a Time-Restricted Feeding regimen, your daily caloric intake might actually be 2500. We will get into this in the following three chapters, where we discuss setting goals and picking the regimen that is right for you.

Summary Points

1. The two main types of Intermittent Fasting are called Alternate Day Fasting and Time-restricted Feeding.
2. The primary benefit of Alternate Day Fasting is that it has been shown to be the fastest way to lose weight quickly and keep it off.
3. The primary drawback of Alternate Day Fasting is that, since one is fasting for the whole day, it may be difficult to stick to and requires great discipline.
4. The primary benefit of Time-restricted Feeding is that studies suggest that it is possibly the most effective way of lowering body fat percentage quickly and confers a host of health benefits, such as the more efficient use of energy and increased insulin sensitivity.
5. There really aren't any primary drawback of Time-restricted Feeding other than it may be difficult to skip breakfast if you're used to eating breakfast every day.

Chapter 3
Setting Goals

Now that you know what Intermittent Fasting is and how it can help you to achieve your goals, it is time for us to figure out what precisely your goals are. Not to beat a dead horse, but what's great about Intermittent Fasting is that it cannot only help you to lose weight (or lower your body fat percentage, if that is your primary goal), it actually improves your overall health, and who doesn't want that?

Let's get right to the point. The biggest indicator of success on a diet is having a clear idea of what your goals are. Other important aspects of this goal-setting agenda are having a plan of how you are measuring those goals and setting a timeline for checking your progress. Setting goals for yourself is an intrinsic part of your plan on any diet. Starting a diet without goals is like paying someone to build a house for you without any system for checking on the progress of that house. Three years later, you are still not in that house. All you have are the foundations and a porch. Why? Because you never had a plan of how you were going to check on progress.

So it's important to set goals, and those can be

literally anything. Maybe your goal is to lose 30 lbs. in the next 6 months. Maybe you're getting older, and you've noticed that, out of nowhere, you've developed a ring of fat around your midsection and you really just want to target that. Maybe you've been eating too much, and you've been feeling lethargic, and you want to feel better. Maybe you've been lifting weights for six years, and you've never been able to see your abdominals, so your goal is visible abs. All of these goals are achievable with Intermittent Fasting; the key is just establishing what these goals are and how you will measure them.

The real first step to setting goals and coming up with an Intermittent Fasting Plan is being honest about where you are right now. This means, for most people, stepping on a scale and weighing yourself. Okay, you know you're big, but how are you going to measure if you are progressing on your diet if you don't know what your starting weight is? Weighing yourself makes it easy for you to keep track of your progress on your diet. Perhaps on day 1 of your diet, you were 315 lbs. Well, it's three weeks later, and now you're at 302 lbs. That's progress, and you wouldn't have known that unless you had actually weighed yourself!

Alright, that was an easy one. Another thing you should do is to calculate your BMI. BMI stands for Body Mass Index, and this is how your doctor measures if you are in the normal weight range for your height, or if you are underweight, overweight, or obese. The BMI actually began as a way for insurance companies to have a general idea of the health status of their potential insureds, and it has been so useful that it has become standard in medicine to calculate BMI to have a sense of where someone's weight puts them on the healthiness scale. You can calculate your BMI yourself, though it would be easier and faster to use an online BMI calculator. BMI is your weight (in kg) divided by the square of your height (in meters). Not square root. Square. So:

BMI = Mass (kg) / [height (m)]2

In American terms, that is your weight in pounds divided by the square of your height (in inches) and the whole thing times 703. So:

BMI = Mass (lb.) / [height (in)]2 x 703

But again, it would probably be easier to use an online BMI calculator. So, now you know your BMI. What now? Well, now you need to know where your BMI puts you in terms of overall health. This is important because there is an association between BMI (along with percentage body fat) and risk for cardiovascular disease and Type 2 Diabetes. A BMI in the range of 18.5 – 25 kg/m2 is considered normal. A BMI below 18.5 kg/m2 is considered underweight. A BMI between 25 kg/m2 and 30 kg/m2 is considered overweight, and a BMI over 30 kg/m2 is considered obese.

So we've tackled weight and BMI as preliminaries to set our goals. What's next? Well, since this book is designed to help anyone who is attempting to use Intermittent Fasting to change their body composition, we really need to divide you all into two camps. No, not opposing sides like the Capulets and the Montagues, or the East Side and the West Side, etc. **We need to figure out if your goal is weight loss or targeted fat loss**. It is important to make this distinction because this will help you decide whether you want to go with Alternate-Day Fasting or Time-restricted Feeding. As we touched on in the previous chapter, Alternate-Day Fasting will usually give fast results, but because this diet focuses on rapid weight loss, it is not the ideal choice for someone who already has a lot of muscle and is trying to target merely their body fat.

Alright, what's next on the list? If you have not already done this, you should make a list of all the changes you'd like to see on your diet: flatter stomach, no more love handles, able to walk up the stairs without getting winded. It can be whatever you want. Remember, the point of this is to help you keep track of your progress on this diet, which you will do by simply monitoring whether or not you have achieved that goal. This is a fun one: consider taking photographs. No, not selfies. The point isn't to take a picture to post on Facebook or Instagram, though you're welcome to do that. The idea is that you want a great visual for your starting point so you can see how you are progressing, visually. Anyone who has dieted before knows that sometimes the changes occur slowly and you may not notice them unless someone points them out to you or you see them for yourself. Honestly, on an Intermittent Fasting regimen, it is very likely that you will see the changes as they are occurring.

There are many "must-dos" before starting any diet, but I think one of the most important ones (and one which I saved for last) is to be realistic. Rome wasn't built in a day, okay? If it had been built in a day, it wouldn't have been Rome. By the time of the fall of the Roman Empire in 476, there was a 1000-years' worth of monuments, as Rome grew and matured throughout its history. In the same way, your body can and will change over time, and there is nothing wrong with that. Your body is your temple, and it will take time and effort for that temple to become what it needs to become.

All right, enough clichés. Suffice it to say that Intermittent Fasting really works, and as long as you stick with it, you will reach your goals. For your convenience, there is a table below which will help guide you in getting ready to start your diet.

Must-dos before starting any diet	Why?
Weigh yourself	How are you going to measure progress on a diet if you do not know your starting weight?
Calculate your BMI	BMI is a general measure of health.
Make a list of the changes you would like to see on your diet	As you progress on your diet, you can monitor whether or not you are achieving your list of items.
Ask yourself if your goal is weight loss or fat loss (preserving as much muscle as possible)	This will help you figure out if you should try Alternate Day Fasting or Time-restricted Feeding.
Consider taking photographs	Nothing measures progress on a diet or workout regimen better than before-and-after photographs!
Be realistic	Honestly, the most important thing to keep in your mind.

Alternate-Day Fasting vs. Time-Restricted Feeding

So you weighed yourself, calculated your BMI, decided that your goal is weight loss, made a list of all the changes to your body you would like to achieve on your diet, took a "before" photograph, now what? Well, now you're ready to pick your Intermittent Fasting diet. That means deciding between an Alternate-Day Fasting or a Time-restricted Feeding protocol. Recall that Alternate-Day Fasting means that you are not eating for 24 hours, while Time-restricted Feeding means that you are eating every day, but your feeding period is during a certain window of the day (like 12PM – 8PM). If you'd like, you can take a hop and a skip back to the previous chapter to jog your memory.

Perhaps the easiest way to decide which type of Intermittent Fasting diet to start is to take two (totally fictional) people and walk them through their process of picking a diet. First is Don. Don is 48 years old, 300 pounds, has never been on a diet before, and his doctor has told him that his BMI is 31 and that he needs to lose 60-80 lbs. to reach a BMI of 26, which would be a vast improvement for him. Don eats 4 meals a day, and after a nutritionist reviewed his meal intake, she told him that he's eating 3500 calories a day and he should aim for only between 2000 and 2500, depending on activity level. Don used to frequent gyms back when Larry Byrd was playing, but he pretty much hasn't been to a gym since then. Don's primary goal is to lose 50-60 pounds in the next year and to feel healthier and better about himself. Well, what should Don do? This is a tricky one. Your first inclination may be Alternate-Day Fasting, as we know that this is a fast, effective way to shed pounds quickly. With Don's situation, where he does not appear to be physically active, eats about 1500 calories above his target caloric intake, and we really are not sure what his state of health is, Time-restricted Feeding may be a better choice for him. In particular, Don may have difficulty starting a diet where he's not eating for an entire day when he's used to not only not exercising, but eating pretty much whatever he wants. An important part of Don's diet will be caloric restriction because we want him to not only lose weight but to get into the habit of eating healthier.

All right, the second person deciding on which type of Intermittent Fasting protocol to start is Vlad. Vlad is a Nets fan, and he's 33 years old. He has been working out for ten years, though he does not consider himself a bodybuilder. He has been told that he is in great shape, but he says that he's "never had abs before." Vlad is interested in general physical health, and he goes to the gym 4-5 times a week, doing a combination of weight training and cardio. He is six-feet tall, 180 lbs., his BMI is 24, and his goal is to shed his abdominal fat by summertime because his girlfriend told him that she's not going to the beach with a guy who has a "Dad bod." Vlad doesn't think he has a Dad bod, but he's used to giving Svetlana what she wants, so he's going to make sure he at least has "visible abs" by the time summer comes around. What type of Intermittent Fasting is right for Vlad? Well, since Vlad's goal is targeted fat loss, rather than weight loss, Vlad should also choose Time-Restricted Feeding, although not for the same reason as Don. We don't know what Vlad's diet or caloric intake is like, but even someone like Vlad (who seems to be starting out relatively healthy) can see significant changes on a Time-restricted Feeding protocol.

Summary Points

1. The most important first step to starting any diet, including this one, is setting goals.
2. Part of the process of setting goals is making an accurate assessment of where you are now, and that includes weighing yourself, calculating your BMI, and possibly taking a "before" photo.
3. Once you have set goals for yourself, you can decide whether Alternate-Day Fasting or Time-restricted Feeding is right for you.
4. Finally, be realistic! Diets often fail because we do not set realistic goals for ourselves and become discouraged.

Chapter 4
Intermittent Fasting for Weight Loss

All right, so you have decided to give an Intermittent Fasting diet a try. Your goal is weight loss, and you were searching for a diet that would help you to lose weight in a reasonable amount of time and keep it off. Your extensive research led you to Intermittent Fasting, and you think it may help you to achieve your weight loss goal. Well, you are in luck because not only will Intermittent Fasting accomplish this goal, it will improve your general health as well. In addition to the benefits of Intermittent Fasting mentioned in the previous chapters, IF also confers these goodies:

Benefits of IF for Weight Loss

Reduced Blood Pressure

Reduced Oxidative Stress

Increased Growth Hormone Production

Increased Cell Repair

Increased Metabolic Rate

Better Glucose Control

These are benefits that you want, whether you are a fitness enthusiast who has been engaged in an exercise regimen for years or someone who is beginning a diet on Day 1. If you are overweight or obese, Intermittent Fasting is truly a great choice for you because it can help you to reduce your blood pressure, increase your metabolic rate, and better control your glucose. All right, I'm done selling the diet. Now it's time to jump right in to how to tailor Intermittent Fasting for you.

In the previous chapter, we met Don, a 48-year old gentleman who weighs 300 lbs., has a BMI of 31, and who would like to lose between 50 and 60 lbs. in the next year. That is a tall order, but it is not impossible on an Intermittent Fasting diet. In fact, IF will not only help Don to achieve his goals but when he goes back to the doctor after six months or a year, his doctor will be pleasantly surprised to find that Don's blood pressure and cholesterol are down, and, if the doctor checks this hormone, most likely his testosterone will have gone up, too, because Don has shed so much fat and we all know adipose tissue has an antagonistic relationship with testosterone. All right, this time I'm really done selling the diet.

Initiating a 16/8 Protocol

Don has decided to start a Time-restricted Feeding type of IF, so the next question is, what exactly does this mean for Don? How exactly is he going to *do* it? Well, the first step here is figuring out what Don's feeding window will be, that is, how many hours of the day Don is allowed to eat. We're going to keep it really simple and choose the most common Time-Restricted Feeding protocol, which is the **16/8 protocol**. Sixteen hours of fasting and eight hours of feeding or eating. This is the most popular protocol for a number of reasons. The first is, for most people, this protocol is not so restrictive that it interferes with your daily life. Yes, it may mean that you are not eating anything before you go to work, but depending on how you schedule your window, you will most likely only be fasting for the first three or four hours of your work day and eating after that. The second reason why the 16/8 protocol is so popular has to do with how effective it is. Dieters who give this protocol a try, even men and women who have been working out for years, have seen significant results in as little as three weeks.

All right, so Don is doing the 16/8 protocol. Now he has to figure out when he will eat. Honestly, this is completely up to Don, though he should take into account the following: what time he gets up in the morning, what time he has to be at work, any part of the day where he is engaged in strenuous activity and may need to have a little extra energy, certain meals or food types that he loves and just cannot live without. Okay, let's say that Don works as a forklift operator in a factory and his shift falls between 7 AM and 4 PM, with an hour lunch break at 11 AM. Don usually gets up at 5 AM, and before he started this diet, he would usually eat a large breakfast at 5:30. Again, keeping it simple, we're going to recommend to Don that his eight-hour window fall between 11 AM and 7 PM, so that way he can make sure to have his first meal during his lunch break. Now we knows that Don is eating from 11AM to 7PM. What sort of meals should he have? Should he have two large meals, three medium-sized meals, two meals and a snack or maybe even one large meal? We're going to recommend that Don have two meals and a snack in between, but below is a table with some ideas (also featuring a calorie estimate for each meal). It is important to remember that the key to weight loss while Intermittent Fasting is the fast itself, less so the calories, so we're not focused on limiting Don's caloric intake as much as other diets would. No, we're not telling Don to have all of his meals and his snack at McDonald's (which does have healthy menu items, by the way), but it isn't necessary to put Don on a 1200 calorie diet that he's going to give up on in the first week because he's starving. Two thousand calories a day is acceptable for Don on his Time-restricted Feeding diet.

Meal breakdown	Suggested Meal times	Total Number of Calories
Two meals a day	11 AM and 5 PM	1600 calories
Two meals and one snack	11 AM and 6 PM (snack at 2 PM)	2000 calories
One meal a day	11 AM	1200 calories
One meal and one snack	11 AM and 4 PM	1600 calories
Three meals a day	11 AM, 4 PM, 6:30 PM	2000 calories

The table above offers suggestions for a beginner just getting started out on IF. The idea is to give you a sense of how you would incorporate a 16/8 Time-restricted feeding schedule into your daily life and the sort of calories you could expect. The reality is that each person deciding to give this diet a try is different. Some of you will have weight concerns and so you have to think about whether you will be able to stick to a diet that is super-restrictive. Again, an advantage of IF is that you do not have to restrict your calories the way that you would in a diet that is based solely on caloric restriction. The long and short of it is, if you know that you can handle 1200 calories a day and you really want to lose weight fast (because your sister's wedding is coming up and you have to get into that bridesmaid dress or that best man tux), fine, you can choose to have one meal a day, or one meal and a snack. But you don't have to. If you'd like to have two meals and a snack, you can choose that and still expect to see dramatic results on this diet.

Okay, so we decide to have Don try two meals and a snack in between because he is new to dieting and we know that he is unlikely to stick to the diet if it represents a drastic departure from what he is used to. Skipping breakfast is hard enough. This diet will give Don 2000 calories a day. Now, you may be thinking, "How is Don going to shed all that fat if he's getting his recommended daily intake of calories and not in a deficit?" Again, Don does not have to be in a caloric deficit in IF because fat loss is being triggered by the six hours, he's up in the morning (from 5AM to 11AM) in which he is not eating.

The next thing for Don to do is to figure out what he's actually going to be eating during his two Meals and a snack because Don is used to eating whatever he wants, and reading labels or knowing how many calories are in this or that is not something that he's ever had to do. Well, first of all, Don needs to get into the habit of reading labels. Let's not beat around the bush on that one. Most Americans have very distorted perceptions of what is a normal-sized portion of food and this is one of the reasons why we tend to overeat. Okay, so Don needs to start reading labels to get an idea of exactly how many calories are in those Reese's peanut butter cups that he snacks on right before bedtime (not a good habit, by the way, and one that Don won't be engaging in anymore since his last meal is at 7 PM!). But we're not going to leave Don hanging out on his own, we're going to help Don by offering some meal suggestions (with recipes) at the end of the chapter.

Monitoring Progress on your Time-Restricted Diet for Fat Loss

We tried to drive this home in the previous chapter, but one of the most important components of your diet will be deciding how you will monitor progress. Are you going to be weighing yourself every week, taking shirtless photos, or what? This is completely up to you, but weighing yourself once a week, at the very least, is a good place to start. Keep in mind that, although IF tends to work rather quickly compared to other diets because eating and losing weight are all hormonally regulated, some people may see weight loss more quickly than others. Some people may even gain a little weight when they first start out a new diet because the body tends to lower the metabolic rate during periods of starvation, especially in people who have a history of binge eating. By binge eating, we mean eating very large meals, sometimes multiple times a day, without any schedule and without any real tie to actual perception of hunger. What's the point here? Yes, weigh yourself at least once a week, but keep in mind that you should commit to a diet for at least 2-3 weeks before you decide to throw in the towel. We don't want you throwing in the towel at all, but we want to make sure you give your diet at least 2-3 weeks before you get discouraged if you are not seeing changes as rapidly as you expected.

Who should try Alternate Day Fasting?

Okay, before we jump into meal suggestions and recipes, we need to spend a moment talking about Alternate Day Fasting, which is the other type of Intermittent Fasting (and one we decided not to recommend for Don). This, naturally, begs the question of who is right for an Alternate Day Fasting protocol. Don is overweight, he needs to lose weight quickly, isn't he the perfect candidate for Alternate Day Fasting? No, he isn't. A major predictor of how effective a diet will be for any particular individual is assessing the likelihood that that individual will stick to the diet. What is the likelihood that Don, a man who is used to eating whatever he wants for more than 40 years, will go an entire day without eating while also maintaining a full-time job? All right, it's not impossible, but not super likely either. We want to choose a diet for Don which will work for him, which will both meet his needs as an individual and which will help him to lose weight.

Who should attempt Alternate Day Fasting then? This is really a good question but isn't an easy one to answer. Someone who is very disciplined and already relatively healthy is the best candidate for Alternate Day Fasting. In other words, if you have dieted or fasted before and you know that drinking only water for a day isn't going to be difficult for you, then you may consider this diet. The other piece of this is that a whole day fast assumes that you are healthy enough to actually not eat for an entire day. Anyone with diabetes or anyone with a condition that affects hormonal balance or that causes significant stress to the body at all should not try this diet. This diet is really for someone who is healthy enough to be able to handle what it will do to the body. Don't get me wrong, people all over the world have engaged in fasts for religious and cultural reasons without any adverse effects. To reiterate, the body is actually designed to handle fasts because the normal pattern of eating for our ancestors would have included (often prolonged) periods of fasting, but most people have some form of disordered eating, often with resulting medical problems, and it may not be a good idea for most people to jump right in to a fast. Remember, we want to pick a diet for you that you will be able to stick to.

Time-restricted Feeding Meal Plans

Two Meals and One snack (to make this into two meals, just cut out the snack)

Meal Number	Meal Name	Dish	Calories
Meal 1	Lunch	Sesame Beef stir-fry with a cup of coffee	700 calories (35 grams of protein)
Snack	Mid-afternoo n snack	Pasta salad with a glass of orange juice	400 calories (20 grams of protein)
Meal 2	Dinner	Balsamic-roasted pork chops (4) with a glass of low-calorie	700 calories (35 grams of protein)

		lemonade	
Totals			1800 calories (90 grams of protein)

Three Meals

Meal Number	Meal Name	Dish	Calories
Meal 1	Lunch	Two Beef Fajitas with a cup of coffee	700 calories (60 grams of protein)
Meal 2	Dinner	Large Protein Salad w/ nuts and beans	500 calories (20 grams of protein)
Meal 3	Supper	Blackened Mahi Mahi Burgers (4) with a glass of low-calorie lemonade	800 calories (80 grams of protein)
Totals			2000 calories (160 grams of protein

Recipes

Sesame Beef Stir Fry

Ingredients	1 lb. flank steak sliced into strips 3 cloves of garlic, minced 1 red bell pepper, sliced 1 green onion, sliced ¼ cup of water 1 tsp. cornstarch 3 tbsp. Kikkoman soy sauce 2 tbsp. brown sugar 2 tbsp. sesame seeds ¼ cup canola or vegetable oil (optional)
Macro Nutrient Breakdown	680 calories 32 grams of Fat 65 grams of Carbohydrates 35 grams of Protein
Prep	- Slice all the necessary ingredients. - Mix soy sauce, sugar, cornstarch, garlic, and onions in large bowl. - Add sliced steak to bowl. - Add all ingredients to frying pan or wok and cook for 5-10 minutes until brown. - Sprinkle sesame seeds and cook for 2 minutes.
Prep Time	20 mins

Blackened Mahi Mahi Burgers

Ingredients	4 4 oz. filets of Mahi Mahi, skin removed 3 cloves garlic, minced ½ tbsp. sea salt ½ tbsp. black pepper 2 tbsp. lime juice 1 tbsp. olive oil 8 leaves of spinach 4 whole wheat buns
Macro Nutrient Breakdown	800 calories 32 grams of Fat 50 grams of Carbohydrates 80 grams of protein
Prep	- Heat grill or oven to medium heat. - Dry filets of Mahi Mahi and set aside. - Rub grill plates or aluminum foil-covered pan with olive oil. - Place Mahi Mahi on the grill or on the pan, grilling each side for 3 minutes. Remove. - Brown the buns, placing on the grill or in the oven for one minute. - Sprinkle the Mahi Mahi with salt, black pepper, garlic and lime juice. - Transfer Mahi Mahi to bun, adding spinach.
Prep Time	10 mins

Chapter 5
Intermittent Fasting for Bodybuilding

If you are a bodybuilder, you are probably familiar with the term IIFYM. IIFYM stands for If It Fits Your Macros, and all this means is that your diet, different from that of someone who is attempting to lose weight, is primarily focused on making sure that you are meeting your macronutrient needs for the day. What a bodybuilder needs calorie and macronutrient-wise is very different from someone who is not spending an hour or more in the gym 4-7 days a week. If a typical man or woman has a recommended daily intake of 2000 calories, of which perhaps 75 grams is fat, 250 grams are carbohydrates, and 50 grams or so are protein, a bodybuilder of about the same size can easily get away with eating 2500-3000 calories in a day. This is partially due to their increased caloric needs related to their workout, but it is also a factor of just carrying around all that muscle.

So what's the point? The point is, if you are engaged in bodybuilding or fitness as a serious pursuit, you will have to tailor you Intermittent Fasting regimen so that you can preserve as much of your muscle as possible while you are shedding fat. This means that you will have to be counting calories and paying attention to your macros. Just like we did in the Setting Goals chapter, you will have to make a good assessment of where you are now, including your physique, and then you will adopt a diet that will help you reach your goal.

Incorporating IIFYM with IF

If you are a bodybuilding and fitness enthusiast reading this, you probably are not only familiar with macros, but you already know what your daily macros are. But let's say that you are not. Let's go back to Vlad, a 6-foot tall bodybuilder who is 180 lbs., has a BMI of 24, with a body fat somewhere between 10 and 20 percent. He is trying a Time-restricted Feeding type of IF because of his girlfriend, Svetlana. Not the best reason to start a diet, but we'll give him the benefit of the doubt. Vlad is familiar with macros and aims to get about 1 gram of protein per pound of body weight, which has been the standard in bodybuilding since at least the 80s, but it's not the only regimen. Some bodybuilding coaches recommend increasing this to 1.5 grams of protein per pound of body weight to account for the grams of fat that you are not eating, and also to encourage the body to preserve and continue to build muscle rather than catabolize it while you're dieting. Some professional bodybuilders are known to eat as much as 2 grams of protein per pound of body weight. Not recommending that, as extremely high protein diets have been proposed as a risk factor for cardiovascular disease and cancer. We're going to recommend to Vlad that he stick to his 1 gram of protein per pound of body weight, which works out to 180 grams of protein. Could that math be any simpler?

What about the other macros? Well, because Vlad was always more concerned with building muscle and never really cared about having super-defined abdominals, he never really cared about his other macros. Since Vlad is being schooled on doing Intermittent Fasting the right way, we will make some macro recommendations for Vlad.

As mentioned again and again in previous chapters, because IF is using meal timing (fasting periods) to trigger weight loss, severe caloric or fat restriction is not critical in this diet as it is in other diets. That doesn't mean that your last meal of the day should be a tub of the least healthy ice cream imaginable. Eating unhealthy, fattening foods is actually a downward spiral that leads to binge eating, so even though Vlad could theoretically be a little lax with his fat and carbs, we want him to start paying attention. Okay, so Vlad's protein is 180 grams, what is the breakdown of his other macros? Well, one thing that bodybuilders need to know, and many of you already do, is that carbohydrates are not your enemy. You actually use carbs for energy. Yes, excess sugar is stored as fat, but we're not super-worried about that, remember? Our fasting is handling this fat situation. So, we're going to say that Vlad will stick to the typical ratio of about 50 percent of his calories for the day from carbs. Of course, Vlad could choose to eat less carbs, but that would mean that he would have to either go up on fats or on protein to reach his daily total of 2000-2400 calories a day. This is basically how IIFYM works. If you go down on one macronutrient, you have to go up on another. So what are we recommending for Vlad?

Vlad's Caloric Breakdown		
Macronutrients	Grams	Calories
Fat	75	675
Carbohydrates	250	1000
Protein	180	720
Totals		2395

Again, this is an imprecise science. If Vlad feels like his carbs are a little too high (now that he's finally paying attention to them), he can actually go down on the carbs to say, 225 grams and increase the protein to 200-210 grams. Or, if he wanted, he could go up a little on the fat. This, in the author's opinion, is the fun part of IIFYM and IF. You can sort of figure out what works for you. Now that Vlad has figured out his macro requirement, he needs to do the same things that Don did in the last chapter. Assuming that he's doing a 16/8 split, he needs to then figure out what his meal breakdown for the day will be. Two meals and a snack in between is always a good choice, because you don't feel like you're fasting all day (as you would if you were only eating one meal), and you also don't feel like you're stuffing your face, as you might if you were trying to squeeze three meals into an eight hour period while working a full-time job or going to school. Let's say Vlad goes to school from 10 AM to 1 PM every day and then works part-time from 2 to 8 PM. As Vlad gets up at 9 AM, a good window for his schedule would be 1 PM – 9 PM so that way, he is eating his first meal after school, but before work. His last meal he would get after he gets off of work, and his snack would be squeezed somewhere in between. So this is Vlad's IF protocol: 16/8 split Time-restricted feeding, 1PM-9PM, Two meals and a snack, 2400 calories a day (180P, 250C, 75F).

All right, so that was Vlad. What about you? Well, you need to follow the same steps that we followed with Vlad.

Steps to Follow	Why
Calculate desired protein intake based on weight	Because protein, duh!
Figure out carbs and fats based on the calories that are left after you've subtracted the protein	Well, you can't live off of just protein, can you?
Choose a split (16/8, 20/4)	When you are fasting is the essence of IF
Choose how you will divide your meals	For practical reasons

The 20/4 Split

Just so that we can pat ourselves on the back for at least discussing this, the 16/8s split (though popular) is certainly not the only split that you can do. Indeed, the author has seen at least one YouTube video advocating for a more severe split, and the 20/4 split would be an example of that. That's four hours of eating and 20 hours of fasting. Naturally, the difficult aspect of this split will be how exactly you will get all of your calories in a four-hour window. Do you spend the whole four hours eating?

It's difficult, but not impossible. It may incline you to binge a little, but guess what, this is pretty much the split that contestants on *Naked and Afraid* do. Why? Because it isn't easy having to hunt all your food yourself when you don't even know how to make a decent spear!

Well, the long and short of it is, you can certainly choose a feeding window less than 8 hours, but this, probably, is not the best option for a beginning dieter who is not accustomed to fasting.

And just because we don't want to leave Vlad, Svetlana, and all the other fitness enthusiasts hanging, we will offer Vlad a recipe, too (on the next page).

Vlad's Muscle Borsht with Beef

Ingredients	1 lb. flank steak cut into cubes 8 oz. mushrooms, sliced 1 tomato, sliced 1 lb. of beets, peeled and shredded 3 cups of cabbage, shredded 2 cups of carrots, shredded 2 cups of onions, chopped 2 cups of celery, chopped 1 cup of red wine 1 cup of tomato sauce 8 tsp canola oil 6 cups of beef broth 2 tbsp. Worcestershire sauce ½ tsp of love for Mother Russia (just kidding)
Macro Nutrient Breakdown	310 calories 12 grams of Fat 26 grams of Carbohydrates 20 grams of Protein
Prep	- Slice and dice the steak, mushrooms, and vegetables while heating 4 tsp of canola oil in a large soup pot to medium heat. - Add about ¾ of steak sliced into cubes to the pot that has been heated to medium heat. Brown steak, frequently stirring, for 3 minutes. Transfer to a large bowl. - Add diced mushrooms along with another 2 tsp of oil to the pot, stirring for about 5 minutes. Transfer to bowl.

	- Add the remaining 2 tsp of oil to the pot followed by the tomatoes, beets, cabbage, carrots, celery, and onion. Cook for about 10 minutes. Add wine. Stir. Add broth, Worcestershire sauce, tomato sauce. Cover and bring to a boil. Reduce heat and cook for another 30 minutes. - Add the remaining steak and simmer for another 2 minutes.
Prep Time	1 hr.

Summary Points

1. Most bodybuilders attempting IF will have to incorporate IIFYM (If It Fits Your Macros).
2. Bodybuilders and fitness enthusiasts should begin by calculating desired caloric intake, followed by breaking down of macronutrients.
3. Choose an IF split, 16/8 is recommended, and then figure out how you will fit your meals into your feeding window.

Chapter 6
Frequently Asked Questions

1. What is the best way to Intermittent Fast?
The best way to Intermittent Fast is whatever way works for you. Whichever type of Intermittent Fast fits your needs and your goals, whether you are talking about an Alternate Day Fasting Schedule or a Time-Restricted Feeding protocol, is what you should choose. Personally, I found a 16/8 split TRF helped me lower body fat very quickly while retaining muscle. This is a split that was popularized on YouTube and other social media outlets and which remains quite popular due to its benefits, which most people experience fairly rapidly.

2. Is Intermittent Fasting safe?

As mentioned in the first chapter, Intermittent Fasting is perfectly safe for most people. Not only is it safe, but it actually replicates the natural eating behavior of our human ancestors. A hunter-gatherer of six thousand years ago, for example, would not have been lying around the savanna or in his or her cave eating all the candy and soda that magically appeared in his or her cave during the night. They would not have had a meal at all until they hunted, fished, or gathered it and then cooked it and ate it, whatever the case may be. In other words, our human ancestors essentially fasted every day.

This means that the human body naturally expects periods of fasting, which is why our natural state as humans is, in general, not to be overweight or obese. Obesity usually reflects either high caloric intake or a metabolic problem, which can be due to a hormonal imbalance. When you are intermittently fasting, you are essentially doing what the human body expects and is designed for, that is, you are having your meal during a particular window during the day and essentially eating nothing outside of that period.

3. Should I do Intermittent Fasting if I am a woman?

Intermittent Fasting is perfectly safe for both men and women. In fact, not only is it safe but all of our human ancestors, whether male or female, would have been essentially on an Intermittent Fasting diet. That being said, certain groups should not fast, in general, and that includes pregnant women, people with any sort of hormonal imbalance, or people with underlying medical conditions. If any of these apply to you, you should talk to your doctor before beginning any diet.

4. Can I drink anything during a fasting period if I am on an Intermittent Fasting diet?

The physiology of Intermittent Fasting requires that you have no caloric intake during the period that you are supposed to be fasting. You can drink water during a fasting period on an IF diet, but that's pretty much it. Other types of liquids, like pre-workout of BCAAs (branch-chained amino acids), are not recommended because even though a particular drink or solution may be reported as having zero calories, any substance that has to be digested by the body may disturb the pattern of fat and glycogen mobilization that Intermittent Fasting is attempting to activate.

There is not a consensus on this issue. Some bodybuilders and personal trainers will drink coffee, tea, etc. for their caffeine rush in the morning though, technically, even coffee and tea have calories. The average 8 oz. cup of black tea has 2 calories, while an equivalent size cup of coffee has 1 calorie. That does not include any additives, obviously, like sugar or creamer. And specialty coffees from your favorite chain will have many more calories, from 60 calories up to 300 or 400, depending on what's in it. So, my advice would be to only drink water when you are fasting, even staying away from zero-calorie drinks.

So, yes, you can and should have water while you are fasting, but most other drinks should be avoided.

5. What about supplements?

As mentioned above, the idea of an Intermittent Fasting diet is that caloric intake during the period of fasting should be essentially zero. Therefore, any supplement that contains calories should be avoided. Things like vitamins are generally all right, but other supplements like fish oil or omega-3 fatty acids, any supplement that is actually a covert food, should be avoided because these would, to a certain degree, have to be digested by the body and therefore you technically would not be fasting if you consumed them. It is strange to think of a supplement as a food. Most of them are not, but technically, some of them should be considered food.

6. Do I have to do 8 hours on 16 hours off schedule or can I start with something else?

The problem with most diets is that people often do not stick to them, especially if the diet is very restrictive or represents a sharp change from how the individual normally eats. The norm for many bodybuilding and fitness enthusiasts is the 16/8 protocol, in which you are eating for eight hours in the day and basically fasting during the other sixteen hours. If you are the sort of person who has a busy work schedule and is used to eating throughout the day because your day is so hectic that you have to eat whenever you can and are often hungry, starting out with this split may, for lack of a better word, represent sort of a hardship for you,.

It might be better for someone who is used to eating 12 or 14 hours in a day or more, to ease into an Intermittent Fasting diet. There is no rule of Intermittent Fasting that says that you have to start out with a 16/8 split or you're off the team. It is perfectly acceptable to tailor the earlier stage of this diet to your body and your needs. If this situation applies to you, you might want to start out with a 14/10 split and after a week or two, or whenever you feel comfortable, switch to a 16/8 split. The important aspect of Intermittent Fasting is that you do not want to be eating at all hours of the day, as this is a major reason why many Americans are obese because they are constantly exposing their body to calories, which are then stored as fat.

The reason why Intermittent Fasting works so well rests in the fast itself –the period in which your body is not eating and what your body does when it's not eating –burning fat!

7. Should I do 24-hour fasts occasionally?

It is not a requirement of an Intermittent Fasting diet that you fast for 24 hours ever. To be perfectly honest, I have practiced Intermittent Fasting for certain periods of time over the years, and I never fasted for 24 hours. Some people like to fast for a whole day to "reset the body," as they believe this period of fasting may allow the body to reset or recharge from our generally unhealthy eating habits in this country of basically eating very processed, carbohydrate-packed foods for prolonged periods during the day. The idea of resetting or recharging the body is not completely made up, as the body does have a sense of normal and abnormal, and this practice of ours, of eating throughout the day, from sun-up to sundown, will be perceived by the body as being abnormal.

So you can absolutely fast for a 24 hour period if you like, as long as you do not have any health concerns that would preclude you from doing that, like diabetes. Is this a requirement of an Intermittent Fasting regimen? Absolutely not.

8. Does it matter what my first meal is during an Intermittent Fasting regimen?

Some diets work by targeting the body's metabolism. That is, they cause weight loss by mandating that the dieter consume foods that would favor the body to increase its metabolic rate, like complex carbohydrates, like oatmeal, or some fruits and vegetables. Technically, with Intermittent Fasting, the important bit is not *what* you are eating specifically, but *when* you are eating it. Intermittent Fasting is just that –a fast – and what you eat when you are not fasting is not an inherent part of the diet.

This is one of the advantages of Intermittent Fasting, that technically you can eat whatever you want when you are during your "eating period." So, if you are on an 8/16 split, in which you are eating for 8 hours in the day and fasting for the other 16 hours, what you eat during the 8 hours is technically not a mandated part of the Intermittent Fasting diet. Now, the caveat to this is that the specific foods that you eat can help you to achieve your goals faster. They might even derail you from your diet if they make you hungry. For example, if your last meal of the day is from 7:30PM - 8PM, it may not be a good idea to have Chinese takeout during this period because this type of meal would not only cause you to remain hungry after you have already eaten but the next morning, as well.

The long and short of it is that, technically, what you eat during the eating period of the diet is not an essential part of the diet. In this book, we encourage you to eat certain types of foods that will help your body to process foods in a healthy, efficient way and also help you to stick with the diet. So though you can technically eat whatever you want during your eating period on an Intermittent Fasting diet, this book suggests certain types of foods to help you in your journey, and recommended meal types and recipes have been provided.

9. Do I have to restrict my carbs while I'm on an Intermittent Fasting diet?

The great thing about Intermittent Fasting is that it is all based on meal timing, so you actually have the freedom to choose what meals you are eating when you are not fasting. Because many diets, like the paleo diet, pay close attention to carbs, some people do choose to restrict their carbs on this diet as well. But it is important to remember that one of the most important aspects of a diet – and a big indicator as to whether you are likely to stick with it – is how well the diet fits into your life. If you are used to eating throughout the day, lowering your carbs AND eating in an 8-hour period may be too overwhelming, and you might be less likely to stick with the diet. So, it might be a good idea to eat healthy when you are starting your Intermittent Fasting regimen, but you do not have to go Beast Mode.

10. Why do some doctors and personal trainers recommend eating every 3 hours, or 5 to 6 small meals every day?

Many health educators suggest eating smaller meals throughout the day, for example, every three hours, because they recognize that one of the major causes of obesity is the tendency for Americans, and other people in Western countries, to consume very large meals, essentially binging on food. This binging overwhelms the body and causes us to store this excess energy as fat. Eating smaller meals throughout the day is designed to prevent us from binging, so our body is not encouraged to store massive amounts of fat.

But, if you are following an Intermittent Fasting diet,

you are replicating the body's natural pattern of having periods when you are not eating (a fast) and periods where you are eating (your eating period). Therefore, the reasons for eating every three hours are bypassed because your body is burning calories when it is not eating, so there is no need to eat every three hours. Now, if you would like to eat every two or three hours, for example, during your eating period you are perfectly welcome to do that.

11. Are there any drawbacks to Intermittent Fasting?

There are downsides to any diet. One of the drawbacks to an Intermittent Fasting diet is that you may feel like you have less energy at first because you were used to eating at any and all times of the day and you may interpret a lack of food or a perception of hunger as being less energetic. In reality, as long as you have energy stores in your body in the form of adipose tissue (fat cells) and glycogen stores, then your body will always have a source of "energy" during periods when you are not eating.

Related to this question is another: "Won't I get hungry if I am not eating?" This question is addressed at the very end of the FAQs.

12. I work out first thing in the morning? How will I have the energy for my workout if I haven't eaten anything?

Good question. You do not necessarily have to eat anything before a workout, whether you are on an Intermittent Fasting diet or not. In fact, some people choose not to eat before a workout because they believe that the lack of food combined with the exercise encourages and enhances the body's ability to burn fat, which is true. As mentioned above (and previously), when you are not eating your body is mobilizing its energy stores in the form of fat and glycogen to ensure that your body meets its energy requirements.

Our body is a well-oiled machine. It needs fuel at all times to operate. That means that even when you are sleeping your body has energy requirements that it meets by utilizing its energy stores, or whatever source of energy, for example, food from a large meal, that you have exposed the body to. The point, of course, is that even when you are not eating, your body has energy requirements that it is meeting. Studies actually suggest that working out while you are fasting encourages your body to meet its energy requirement naturally, through fat oxidation. So, technically, you do not have to eat before a workout and your body not only can meet its energy requirements, but it is doing it in a healthy, natural way.

13. Is it hard to stick with an Intermittent Fasting diet?

Sticking to any diet can be difficult. Typical problems encountered with a person who has never done IF before is that you may feel weird not to eat breakfast or to not eat right before bed, which many people may be used to doing. It all depends on whether you schedule your meals more towards the beginning of the day versus later in the day.

14. Oh yeah, when should *I have my meals?*

It is completely up to you, as long as you stick to the schedule: 10 AM – 6 PM, 1 PM – 9 PM, etc. Intermittent Fasting gives you the freedom to choose when you would like to have your meals.

15. I am a bodybuilder. Will Intermittent Fasting affect my ability to build muscle? Will I lose muscle if I am on an Intermittent Fasting diet?

This is a major concern of many bodybuilders, or any person attempting to change their life and appearance by building muscle. The bodybuilding and fitness industry is packed with information that seems to suggest that bodybuilders need to be consuming massive amounts of protein during the day, for example, 1.5 grams of protein for every pound of body weight, etc. There is also a belief that a bodybuilder should have certain types of meals after a workout, such as a meal very high in protein. Although there is obviously a link between protein intake and the ability to build muscle, as amino acids are its basic building block, studies suggest that many presumptions regarding protein intake and bodybuilding are not true.

For one thing, studies have suggested that diets excessively high in protein may be connected with increased risk for cardiovascular disease and some types of cancer. This is a very taboo subject in the bodybuilding industry, as it is pretty much accepted by everyone that you need to be consuming large amounts of protein to build muscle. The important thing to note here is that there is moderation in everything, or there should be. Certainly, a bodybuilder training 5-7 days a week would probably have greater protein requirements than someone who is not training at all, but evidence suggests that common beliefs in the industry about how much protein we should be eating may be excessive and unfounded.

The other myth to debunk is an important one: that you need to eat protein immediately after a meal. Now this is a myth that I have personal experience with because, when I was a college student, a friend of mine who was a nutrition major and who, coincidentally, ended up being valedictorian of the college (true story), made it very clear that studies suggest that when it comes to meeting nutritional requirements, the important factor is quantity during the day, not timing. In other words, the key factor to protein intake is actually *how much* protein in a day, not *when* in a day. Again, this does not necessarily mean eating half a buffalo every day to get your 480 grams of protein, but the point is *when* you are getting that protein does not appear to be a key factor.

In terms of a bodybuilder losing muscle while they are on IF, the reality is that every diet carries with it the risk of losing muscle, which is something that all bodybuilders know. This is the main reason why bodybuilders tend to have a "Bulking Phase" and a "Cutting phase." The Bulking Phase is your time to pack on as much muscle as possible, usually by eating above your caloric requirement, while the Cutting Phase is basically your dieting portion. So, yes, chances are that you may lose a little, weeny bit of muscle while on IF, but that would be true of any diet.

16. Is Intermittent Fasting the same as IIFYM?

This was touched on in Chapter 5. IIFYM stands for

If It Fits Your Macros and this has been a popular dieting term in the bodybuilding world for at least the last eight years. Macros just means macronutrients – protein, fats, and carbs – as contrasted with micronutrients, which would be things like vitamins and minerals, healthy oils, etc. Essentially, IIFYM is a regimen of carefully breaking down your daily requirements of protein, carbohydrates, and fats and closely following the regimen. So if your "macros" are 200 grams of protein, 300 grams of carbs, 50 grams of fat, then you would carefully prepare your meals and read your food labels to make sure that you are meeting these requirements.

Is IIFYM the same as IF? No, it is not. Some people may consider Intermittent Fasting to be a type of IIFYM or a sub-class of IIFYM, but Intermittent Fasting does not require you to eat any particular foods, so in this way, it differs from IIFYM. They may overlap, due to how your Intermittent Fasting diet is being tailored, but they are not one and the same.

17. I am a diabetic. Should I follow an Intermittent Fasting diet?

Diabetics have difficulty processing sugar in the form of glucose because they either lack insulin completely, or their body has become insensitive to it. This means that diabetics are at risk of becoming hyperglycemic, hypoglycemic, or ketoacidotic. For these reasons, Intermittent Fasting may not be for you as there will be periods in which your caloric intake is low. That being said, there are diabetics that have tried IF and have experienced success with it.

Any diet may pose a risk for a diabetic, so diabetics

should always consult their physicians before starting any dieting regimen.

18. And last, but not least: Won't I get really hungry if I am only eating for 8 hours a day?

Intermittent Fasting isn't easy. No diet that really works is. In fact, very little in life that's worth having is easy. As you have already seen, a typical IF diet consists of having your meals during a 8-hour window while fasting during the other 16 hours. For some people, that will mean beginning their first meal at 10 AM and having their last ounce of food before 6 PM. Or not eating their first meal until 12 PM and having their last meal before 8 PM. If you have to be at work by 8 AM and you are not eating until lunch at noon, chances are you will be hungry by the time you have that meal, especially when you're first starting out and your body is used to eating at all hours of the day.

Yes, you will be hungry, especially if you have never intermittently fasted before. That's actually the point. During these periods of hunger, your body is mobilizing stores of fat for energy in the form of fatty acids broken down from fat. The mobilization of these fat stores is how your body can meet its energy stores when you are not eating. This is not unusual. As mentioned in the first chapter, and in one of the previous questions, this is not only perfectly safe, but it actually replicates the natural behavior of our human ancestors and most members of the animal kingdom. Most of our animal cousins are not lying around eating all day.

Conclusion

Intermittent Fasting: Complete Beginner's Guide To Lose Weight, Burn Fat And Stay Healthy Through Intermittent Fasting introduced you to the benefits of Intermittent Fasting and provided you with the tools needed to begin your IF diet. You learned that Intermittent Fasting is completely natural and effective as it replicates the natural functions and processes that the human body is designed to undertake.

Intermittent Fasting can trigger both total weight loss and targeted fat loss, while also reducing cardiovascular risk, lowering blood pressure, reducing oxidative stress, improving neurological functioning, increasing release of human growth hormone, and lowering insulin resistance. The most common type of Intermittent Fasting involves eating during a certain period of the day, the feeding window, and fasting the rest of the day. This type of IF is recommended for most people, and it has been shown to cause a significant fat loss in as little as two to three weeks away.

We hope that most of your questions will have been answered in the Frequently Asked Questions portion of this book, and so we feel that you are well-prepared to begin your diet. We hope you enjoyed reading and we wish you the best of luck on your diet!